COLOR EMPOWER MANIFEST

A Coloring Book to Empower Your Dreams

HarperCollins books may be purchased for educational,
business, or sales promotional use. For information please
email the Special Markets Department at SPsales@
harpercollins.com.

First published in 2023 by
Harper Design
An Imprint of HarperCollinsPublishers
195 Broadway
New York, NY 10007
Tel: (212) 207-7000
Fax: (855) 746-6023
harperdesign@harpercollins.com
www.hc.com

Distributed throughout the world by
HarperCollinsPublishers
195 Broadway
New York, NY 10007

ISBN 978-0-06-329999-3

Printed in China
First Printing 2023

Conceived, designed, and produced by
The Bright Press, an imprint of Quarto Publishing plc
Publisher: James Evans
Editorial Director: Isheeta Mustafi
Art Director: James Lawrence
Managing Editor: Jacqui Sayers
Senior Editor: Joanna Bentley
Design: Studio Noel
Cover design: Emily Nazer

FSC MIX Paper from responsible sources FSC® C016973

CREDITS

Unless otherwise stated, all images in this book have been compiled by Studio Noel.
Shutterstock: aliaksei kruhlenia, Anastasiia Veretennikova, Angry_red_cat, Antonov
Maxim, Arina Gladyisheva, barberry, Bluehousestudio, Dasha Kurinna, Designer
things, ekosuwandono, Evgenia.B, fajarrabadi, Franzi, Gizele, GoodStudio,
hadkhanong, Idea Trader, intueri, IrinaOstapenko, IrynaLu, Julia Lullula, Juliana
Brykova, kareemov, Kalinin Ilya, Kotkoa, Len.OK, Letters-Shmetters, Light-Dew,
Luis Line, lunokot, Madiwaso, Marish, Martyshova Maria, Marynova, Masha Dav,
Mashaart, Mashoid Studio, MehediTech, MIX of ALL SOLUTIONS, Motorama,
Neti.OneLove, oleskalashnik, Oxy_gen, Paragorn Dangsombroon, robin.ph, scops_
art, StockSmartStart, Studio77 FX vector, Sudowoodo, Suwi19, sweet kiwi, Tartila,
Tatyana_zenart, TopVectorElements, Valentina Antuganova, Vasya Kobelev, venimo,
VikiVector, Yana Malyanova, Yayayoyo, YuHusar.

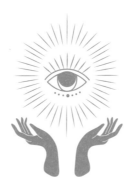

COLOR
EMPOWER
MANIFEST

A Coloring Book to Empower Your Dreams

Lona Eversden

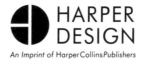

HARPER
DESIGN

An Imprint of HarperCollins Publishers

CONTENTS

This book brings together images and words, specially designed and written to bring clarity and potency to your manifestations. Flip through the book to find the topic you want to focus on, or use the thumbnails below as a visual guide to help you choose the perfect artwork for your mood.

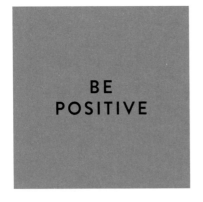

BE POSITIVE

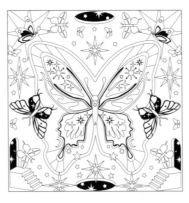

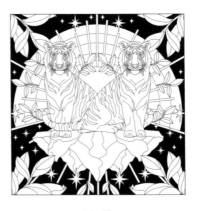

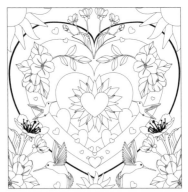

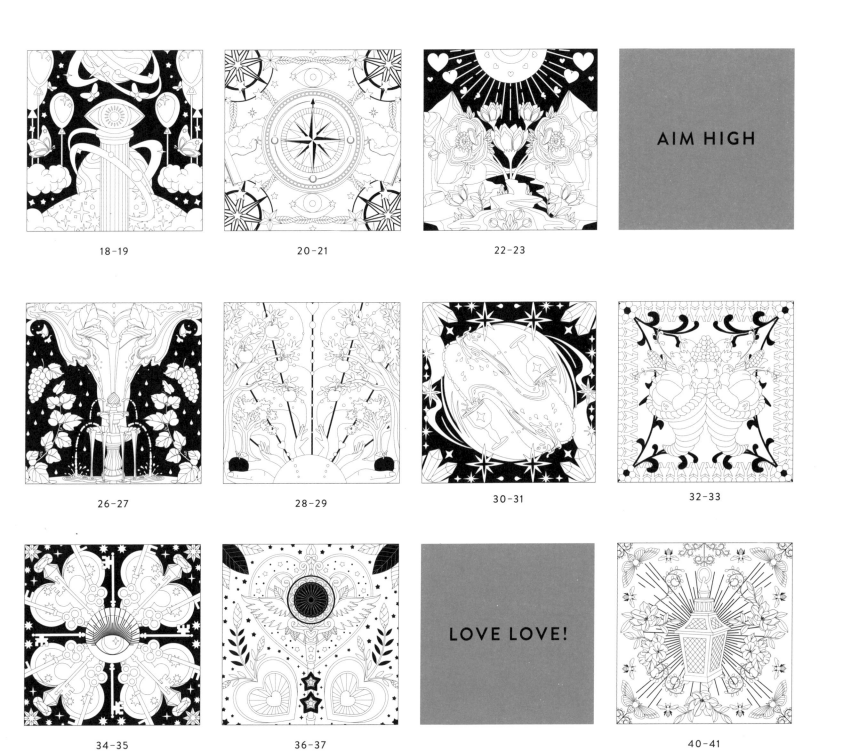

18–19

20–21

22–23

AIM HIGH

26–27

28–29

30–31

32–33

34–35

36–37

LOVE LOVE!

40–41

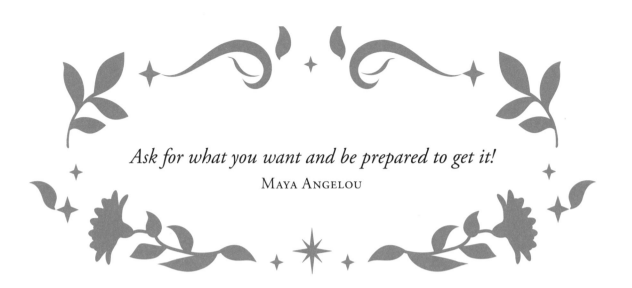

Ask for what you want and be prepared to get it!

Maya Angelou

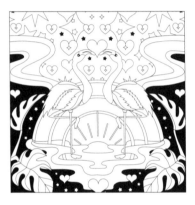

42–43

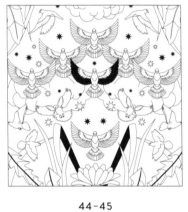

44–45

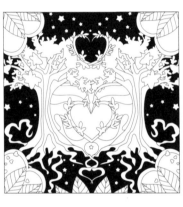

46–47

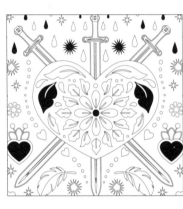

48–49

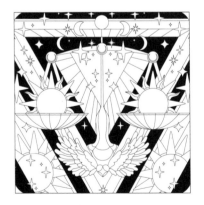

50–51

EMPOWER
YOURSELF

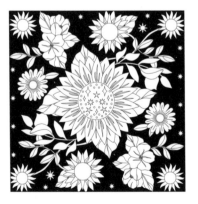

54–55

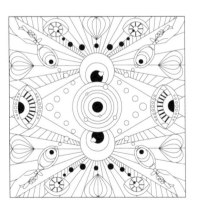

56–57

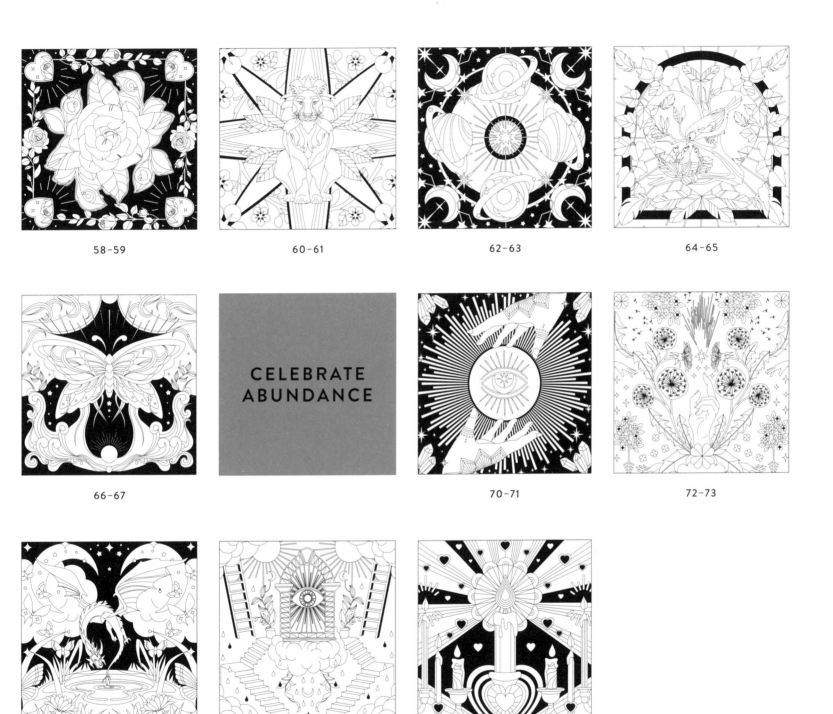

58-59

60-61

62-63

64-65

66-67

CELEBRATE
ABUNDANCE

70-71

72-73

74-75

76-77

78-79

INTRODUCTION

You may be drawn to this book because you already know about manifestation and are interested in learning new ways to practice it. Perhaps you have discovered the wonderful effect coloring can have on your mood and are keen to use it in a more purposeful way. Or maybe you were gifted this book by someone who cares about you. No matter how these pages came to you, they are an invitation to use coloring to manifest your way to a happier, more fulfilled you.

HOW TO MANIFEST

Manifestation is based on the idea that we can attract what we want into our lives through positive thought, faith, and affirming actions. It's the art of breathing life into your dreams and turning them into reality.

There are many ways to practice manifestation, and all of them begin with the foundational principle of knowing what you want. Why is that so important? Because it's only when you are absolutely clear about what you are trying to achieve that you can focus your mind on it and commit to making it a reality.

Once you know what you want, you need to ask the universe for it. The simplest way to do this is through affirmation: positive statements that are presented as

if the goal is already in sight. Some people write their affirmations down each morning and evening. Others use them like a mantra as they go about their day. Still others like to work creatively, through a vision board or painting. It's often useful to combine words and images, as in this book with its specially designed illustration for each affirmation.

Being clear about our goals can sometimes be enough to bring them to fruition. But manifestation usually involves a call to action—so think about whether you are behaving in ways that align with your dreams and commit to taking any steps you can to move closer to your goals. If you want to increase your friendship circle, for example, ask yourself how much you are talking to people as you go about your day, reaching out to new contacts, and accepting invitations that intrigue you. Think more generally, too, about the energy you are putting out into the world. If you want to bring more love into your life, send loving energy outward. If you want more money, then notice and be thankful for the money you already have.

Manifestation is a two-way process, a balance between receiving and giving, believing and doing. It requires trust in the process, however quickly or slowly things may seem to be unfolding. You may not get exactly what you want right away, but acknowledge and feel gratitude for anything you do get, believe in the universe's capacity to provide, and commit to doing whatever is in your power to create the life you want.

COLOR YOUR DREAMS

Coloring is a proven way to release stress and combat negative thinking, so it can act as a gateway to the positive mindset we need to help us achieve our goals. Each coloring project in this book has been created to reflect the affirmation that it accompanies. Spend some time contemplating which page you want to work on. You'll find thumbnails of all the images in the table of contents, so take a look and see which draw you in, or flip through the book until you find a page that resonates.

Before you start coloring, read the affirmation out loud or repeat it in your mind several times. Notice any feelings or thoughts you have in response, and think about whether this is a goal you can believe in and commit to; if it doesn't feel right for you at this moment, follow your instinct and choose a different page to color.

Once you have found an affirmation that resonates with you, allow the simple act of coloring to clear your mind and release any stresses or anxieties you have. As you color, pause from time to time—perhaps whenever you change your pen or pencil—and restate the affirmation.

MATERIALS

Felt-tip pens or colored pencils are all you need to complete the designs. You may like choosing colors that fit the affirmation as well as the image: calming blues and greens for peaceful affirmations, pinks and reds for those concerned with love, energizing oranges or yellows for goals connected with work and focus. Or you may enjoy picking the colors that speak to you at the time.

Parts of each image are printed with metallic ink to illuminate the pages and reflect the preciousness of your dreams. These areas can't be colored, but you can choose shades that complement them or perhaps use your own metallic pens to match.

There is no wrong way to color the illustrations: what works for you is best. Have faith in your choices and have faith in the power of positive manifestation to turn your dreams into reality.

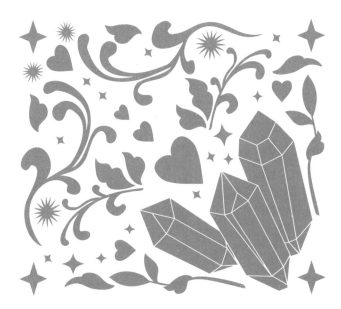

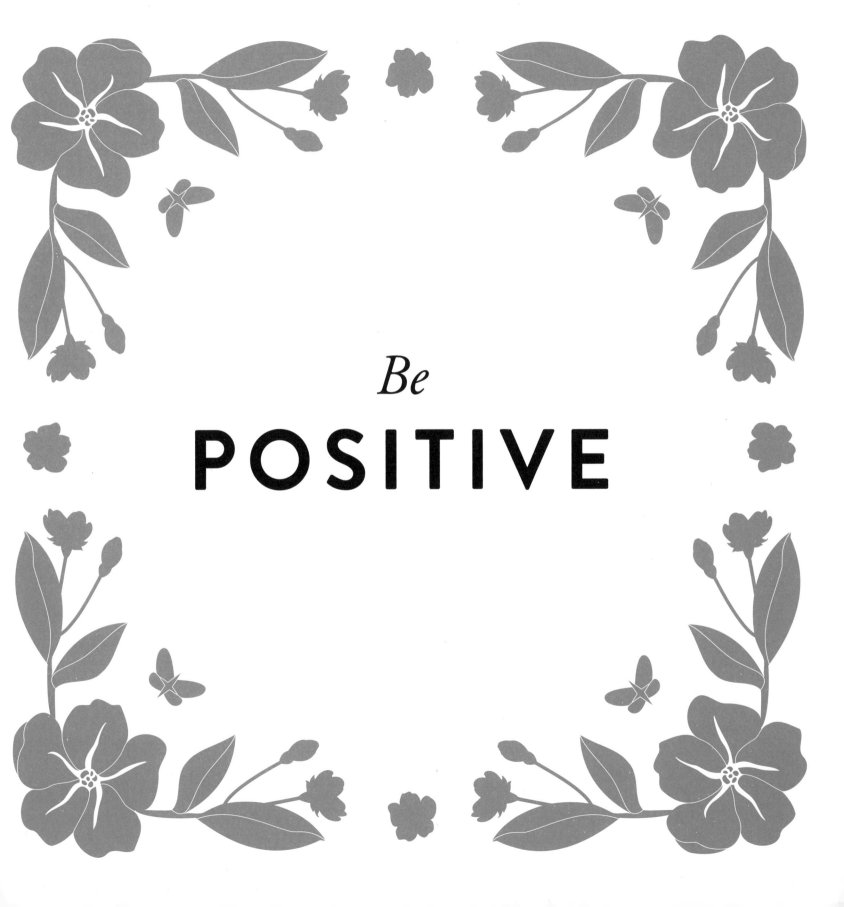

Be
POSITIVE

*Thank you, universe,
for showing me that I am
unique, lovable, and valuable.
I'm so grateful that I have
the courage to follow my own
path, no matter what
others are doing.*

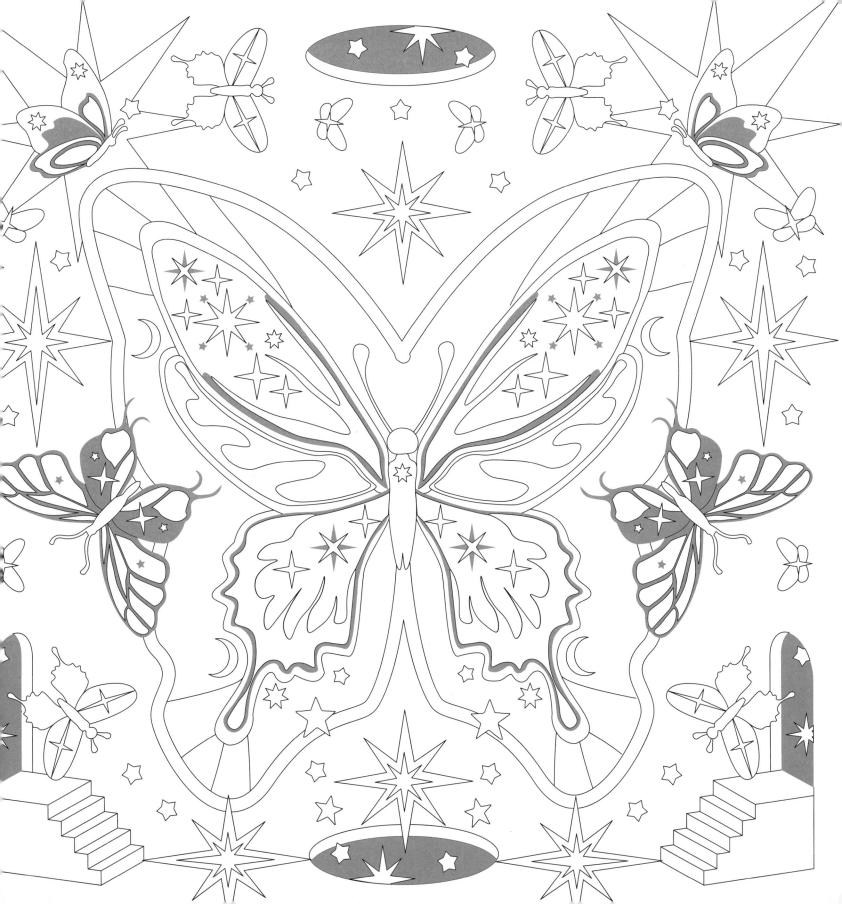

*I am growing
more and more confident,
trusting that I can handle
whatever the day brings
and turning challenges
into opportunities.*

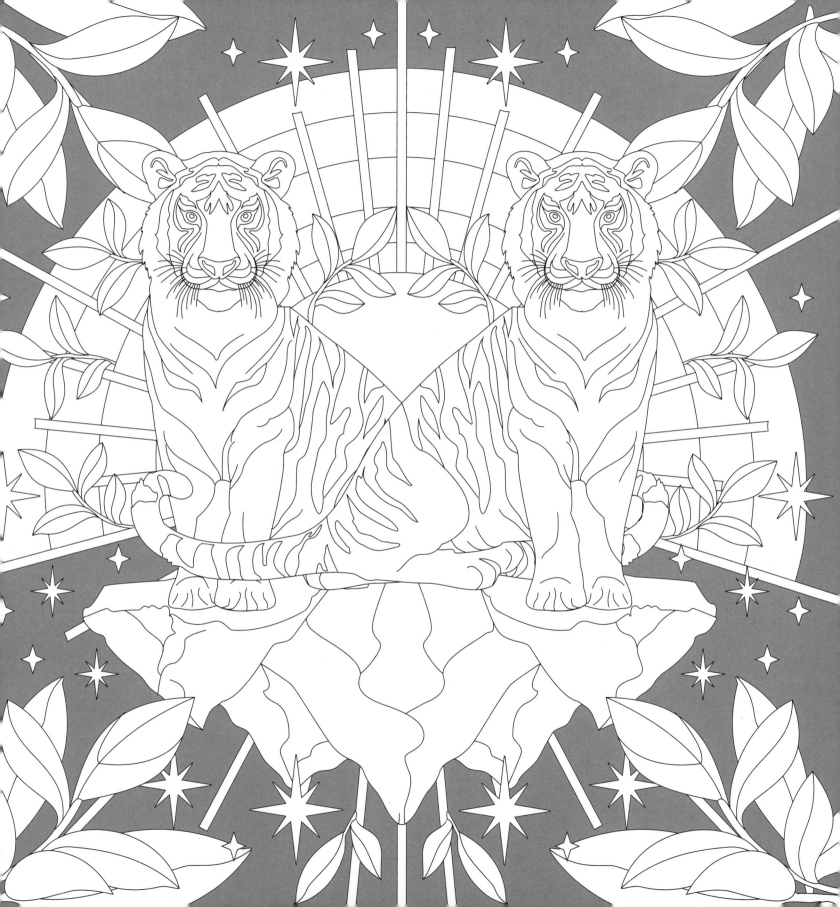

*Positivity comes
naturally to me.
I use positive thinking
to manifest success
and happiness.*

It's becoming easier for me to rise above anxiety. I love how I can always draw on a sense of inner calm and joy and let go of worries.

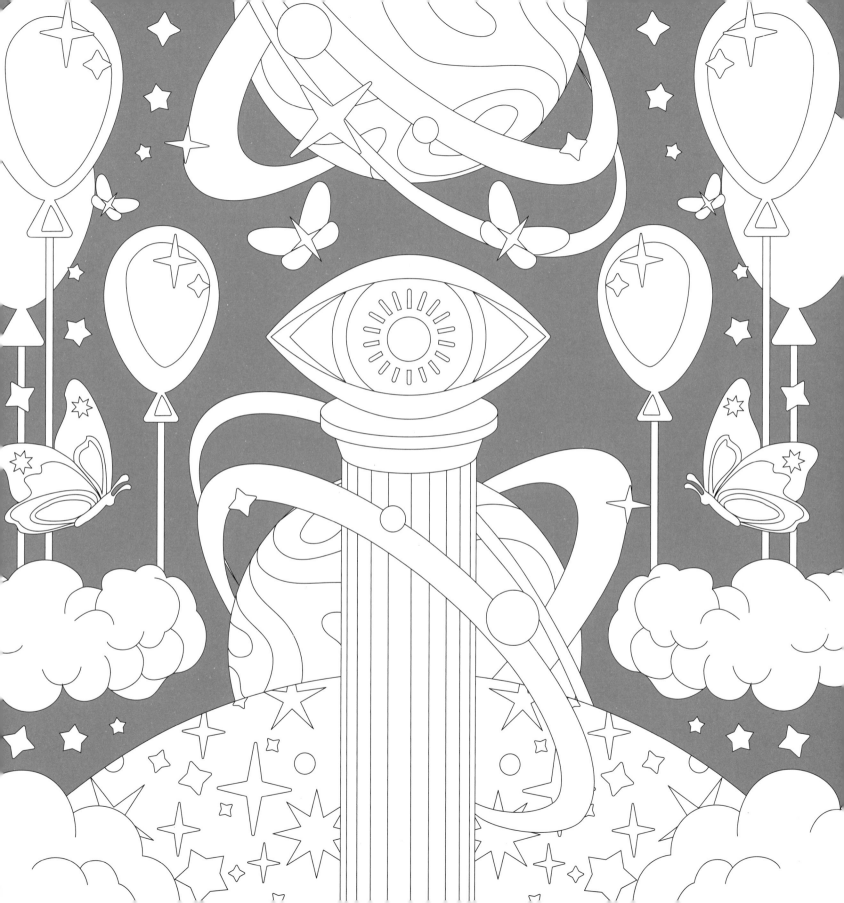

*I navigate where I am meant
to be and trust that I have all
the qualities and skills to manifest
the future I want. I have an inner
wisdom that helps me to know when
I am turning in the right direction.*

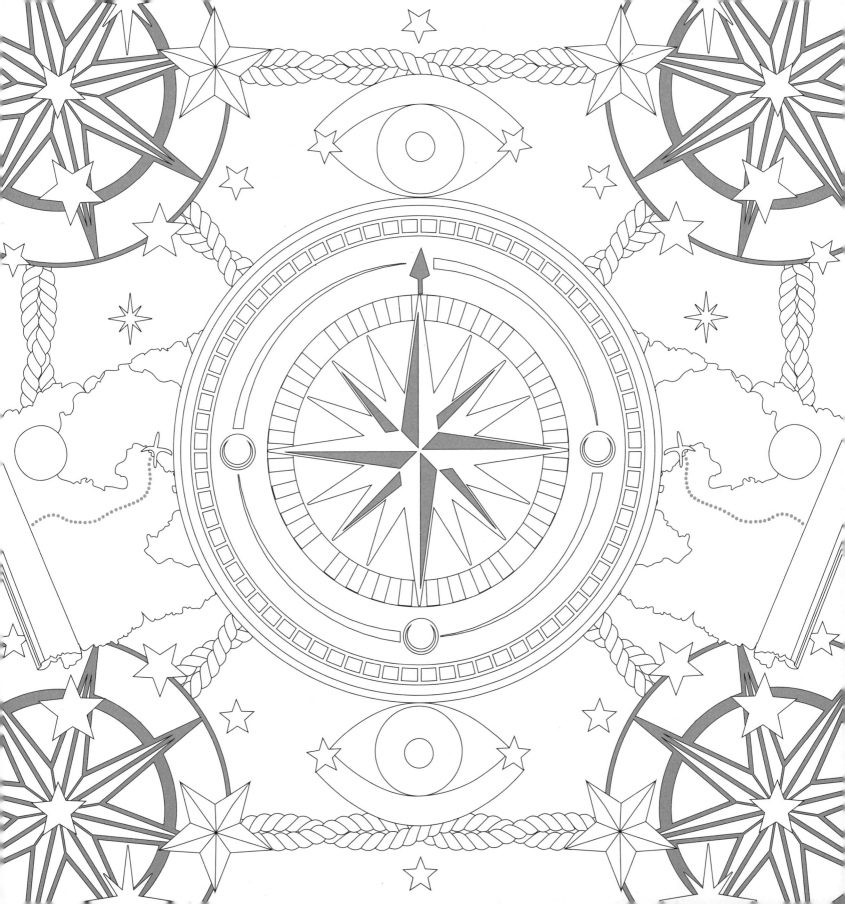

Something wonderful happens to me every day. When I look around, I notice small ways the universe is smiling on me. Today I will see signs of love and beauty wherever I go.

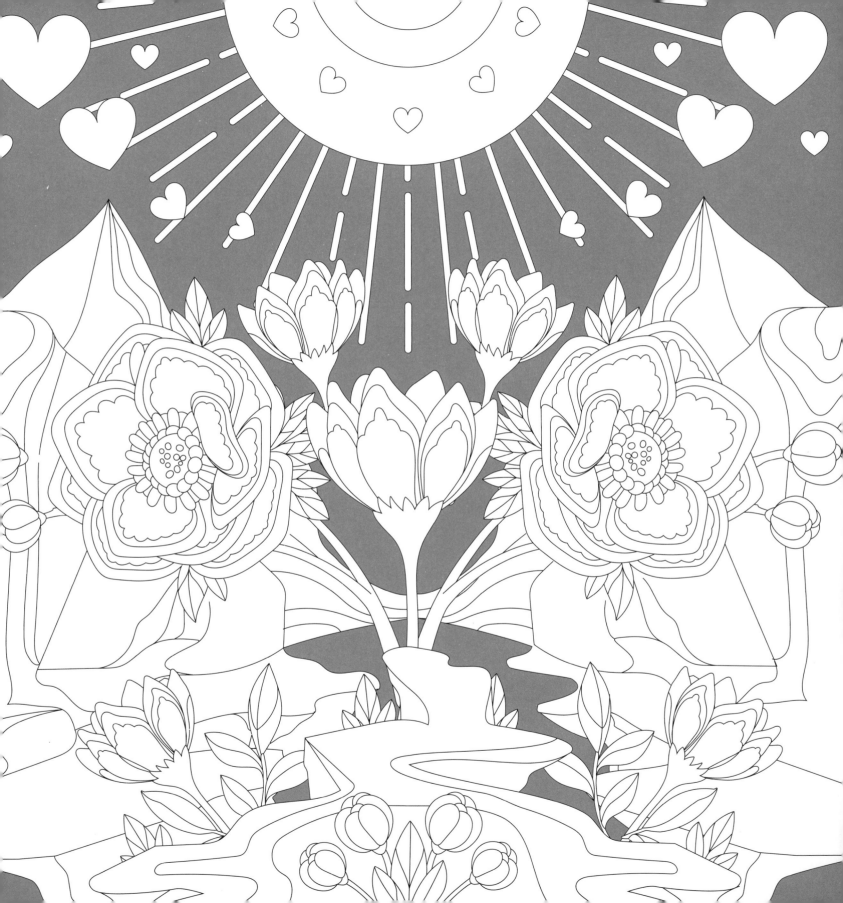

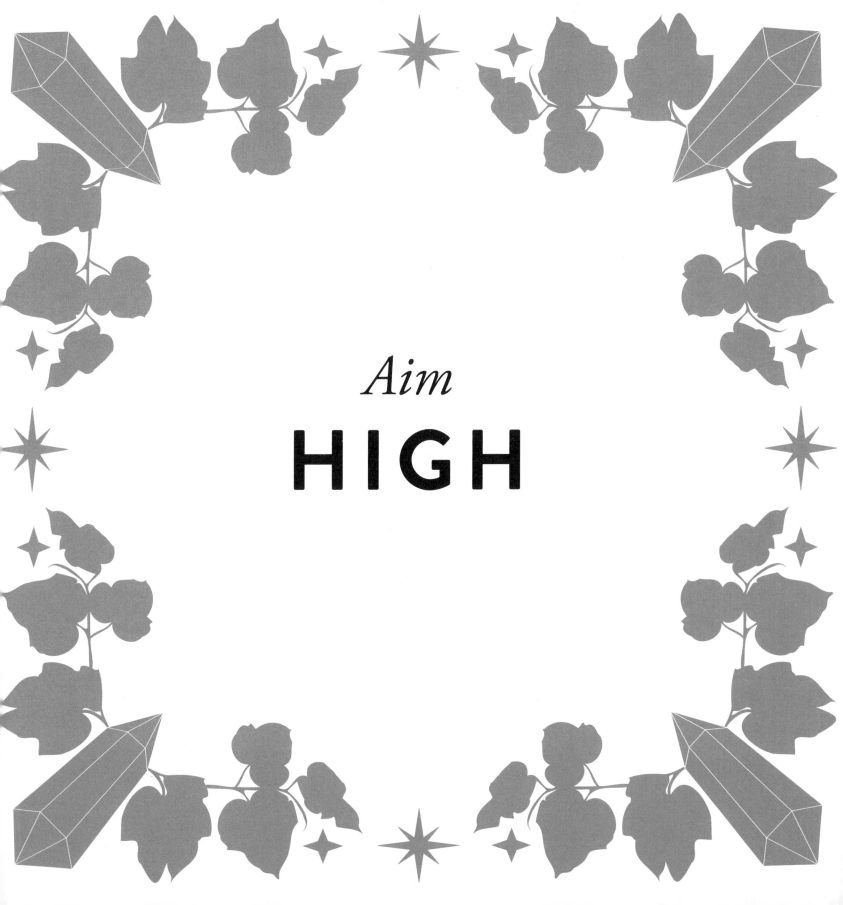

Aim
HIGH

*Money flows easily
and effortlessly into my life,
and I welcome it
with thanks.*

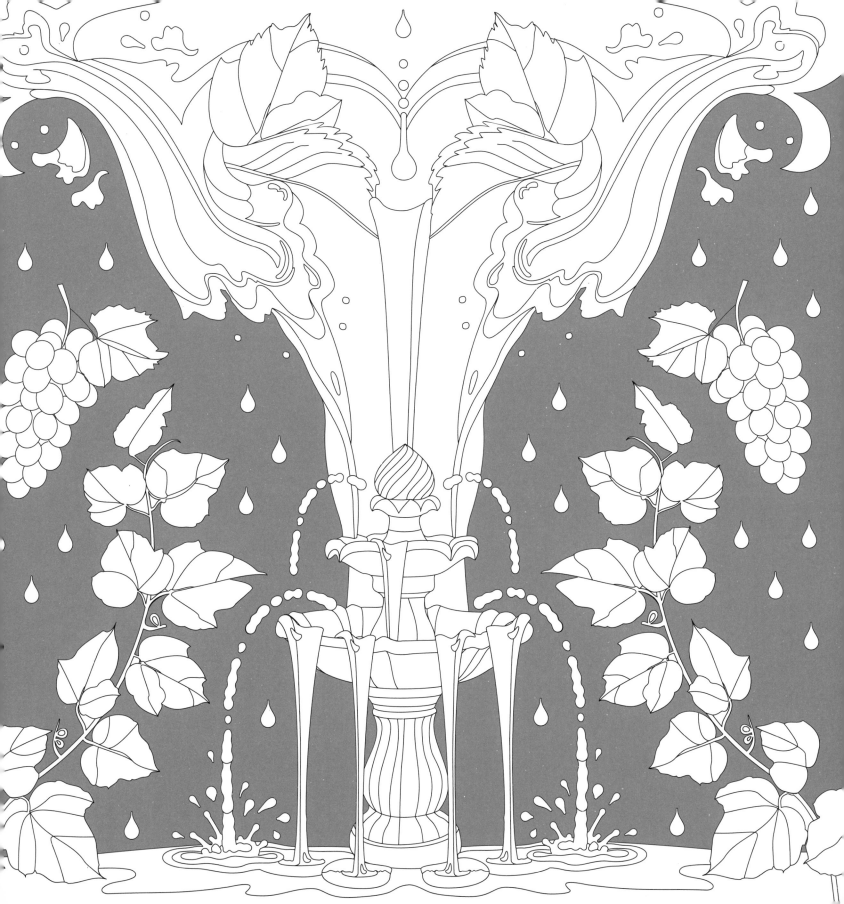

*My career is unfolding just
as it should. It gives me everything
I need to grow as a person as well
as all the financial rewards I deserve.
I trust and value my coworkers
and feel supported by them
in our joint endeavors.*

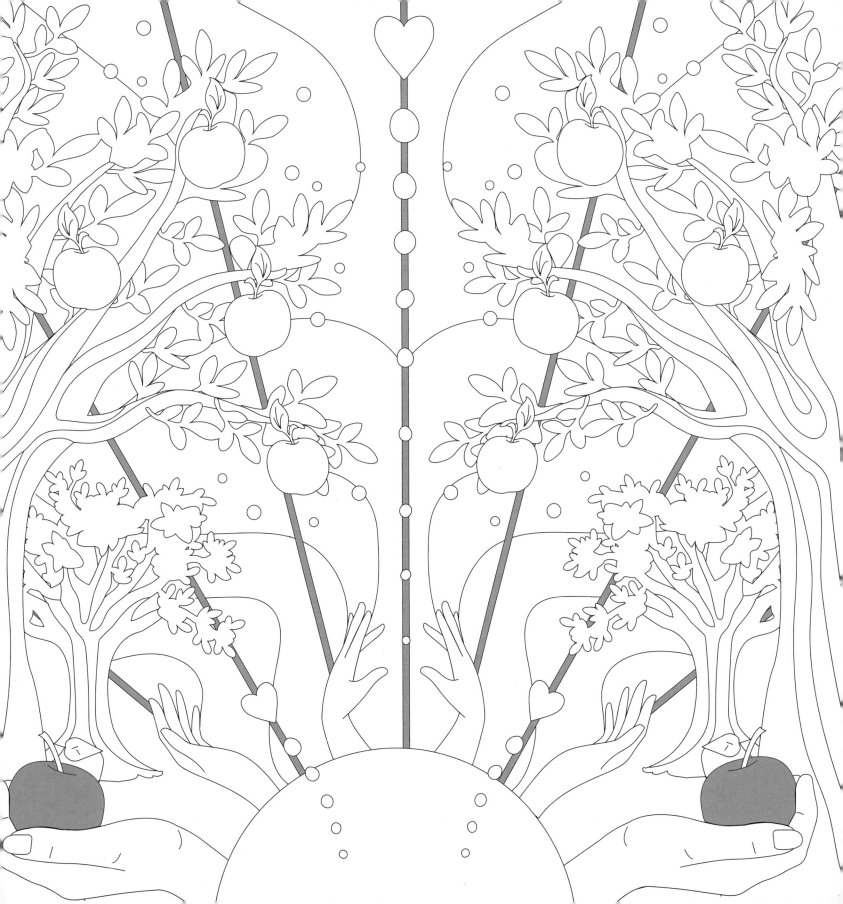

The more I give to others,
the more I receive back.
Gifts come to me in expected
and unexpected ways.

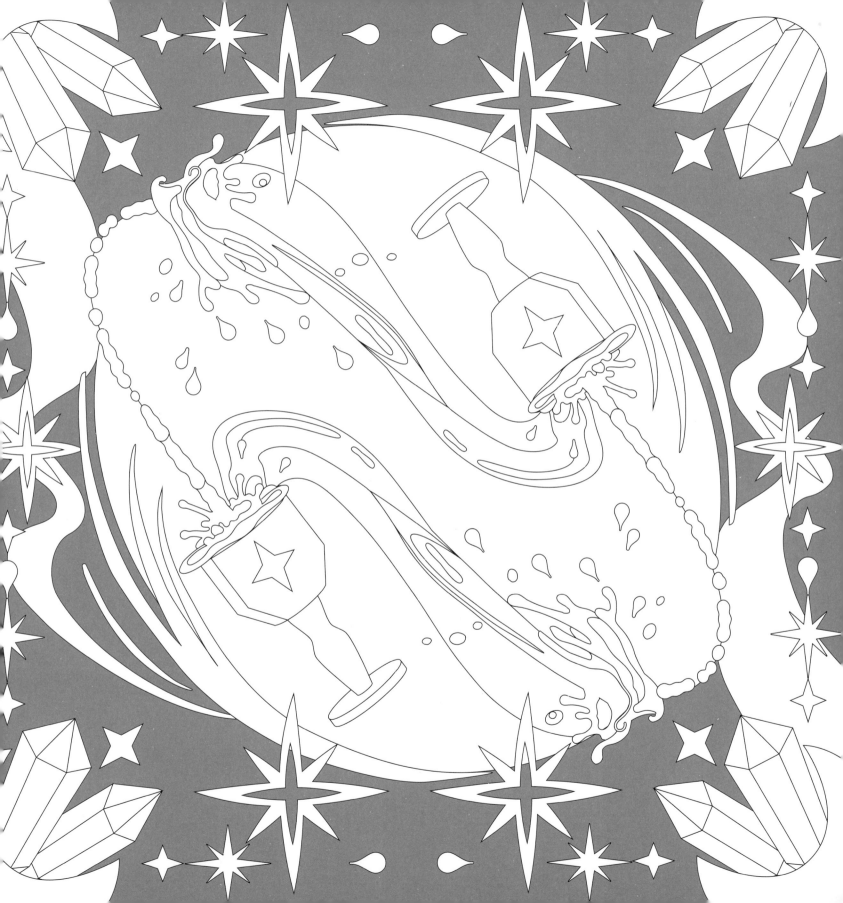

*There is abundance
in all areas of my life.
It doesn't occur to me to compare
myself to others. I know there
is enough for everyone and I can
enjoy the achievements of friends,
colleagues, and family as well
as celebrate my own.*

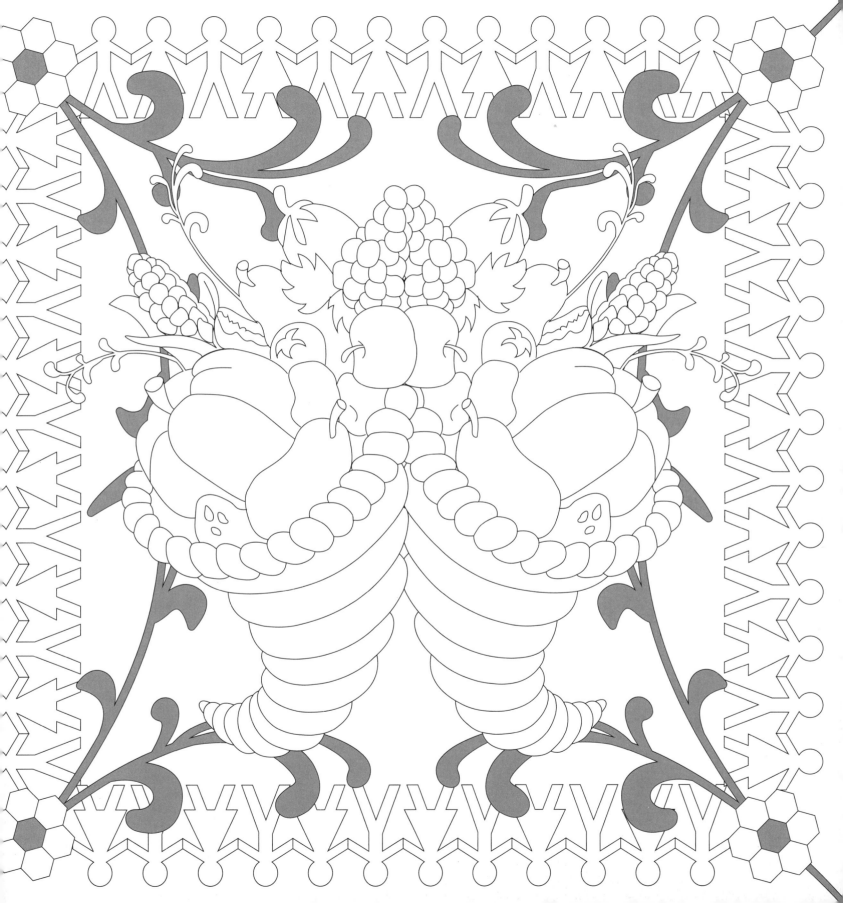

The great things I deserve
are coming my way. I get what
I want because I recognize
my desires and focus on whatever
I seek, whether it's a promotion
or a pay raise or time off.
I hold the key to my own success.

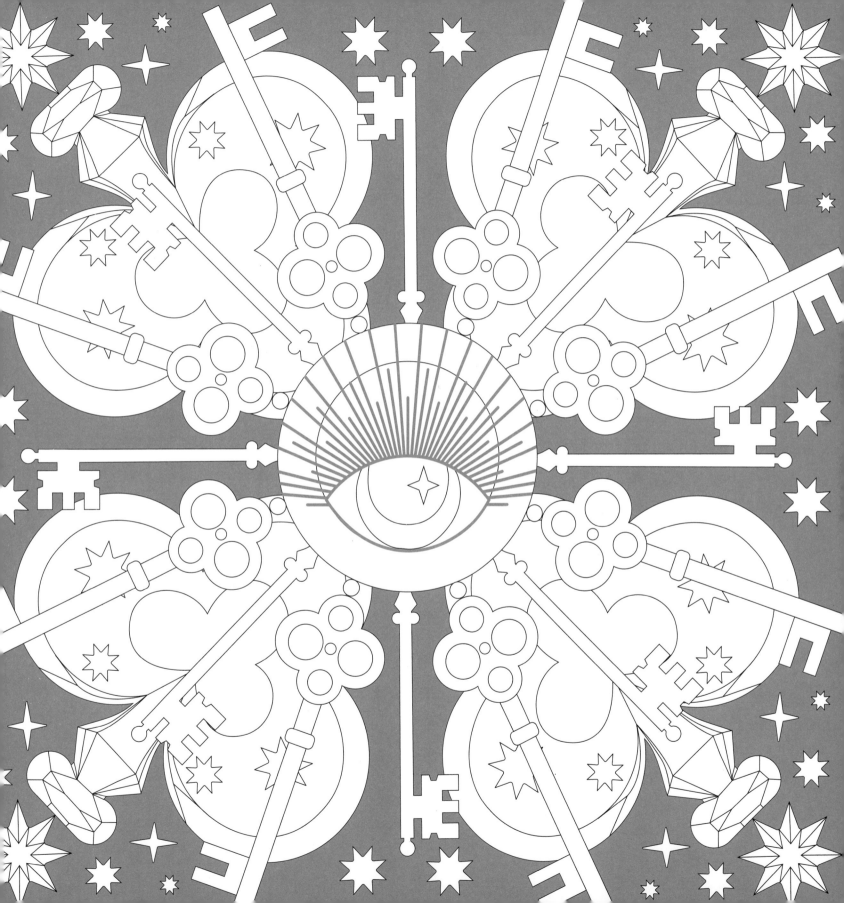

I am a magnet attracting worthwhile people who can help me progress. I find networking enjoyable and I give each person I meet my full attention to allow them to see my best self, trusting that good things are coming.

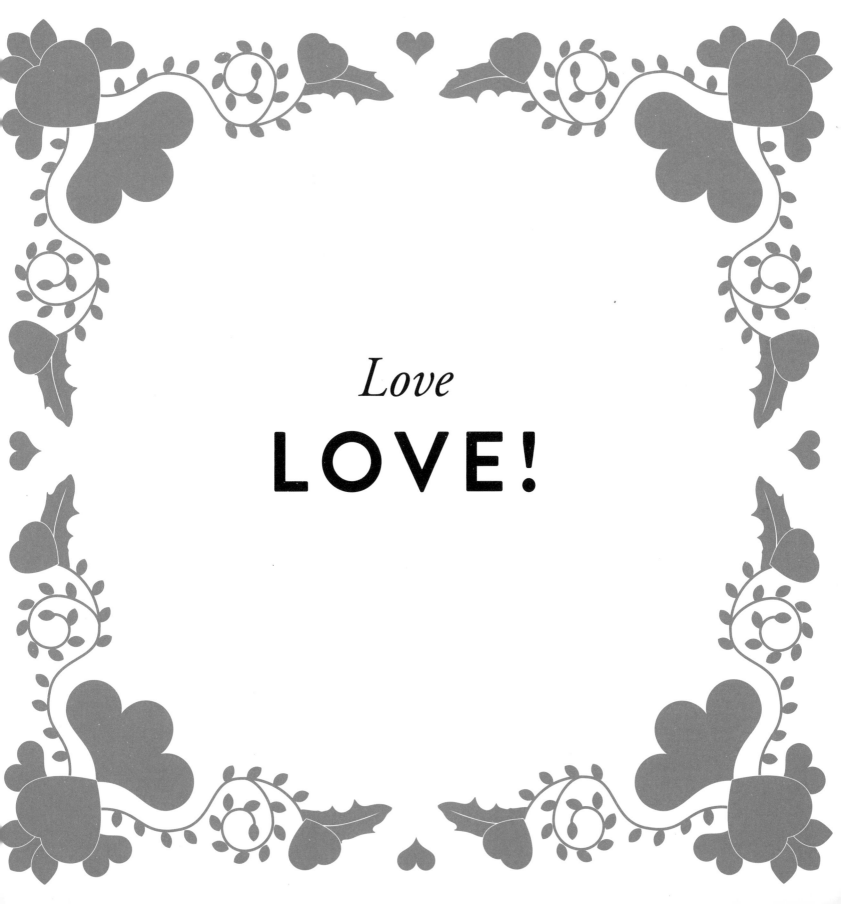

Love

LOVE!

Social situations allow me to shine. I radiate confidence, attracting people with good intentions toward me and sending good vibes to all.

*My heart is open to a happy
and healthy relationship.
When I search for my perfect partner,
I look past the surface and can see true
love ready to be shared. I know that
I am worthy of love and feel ready
to receive and give it.*

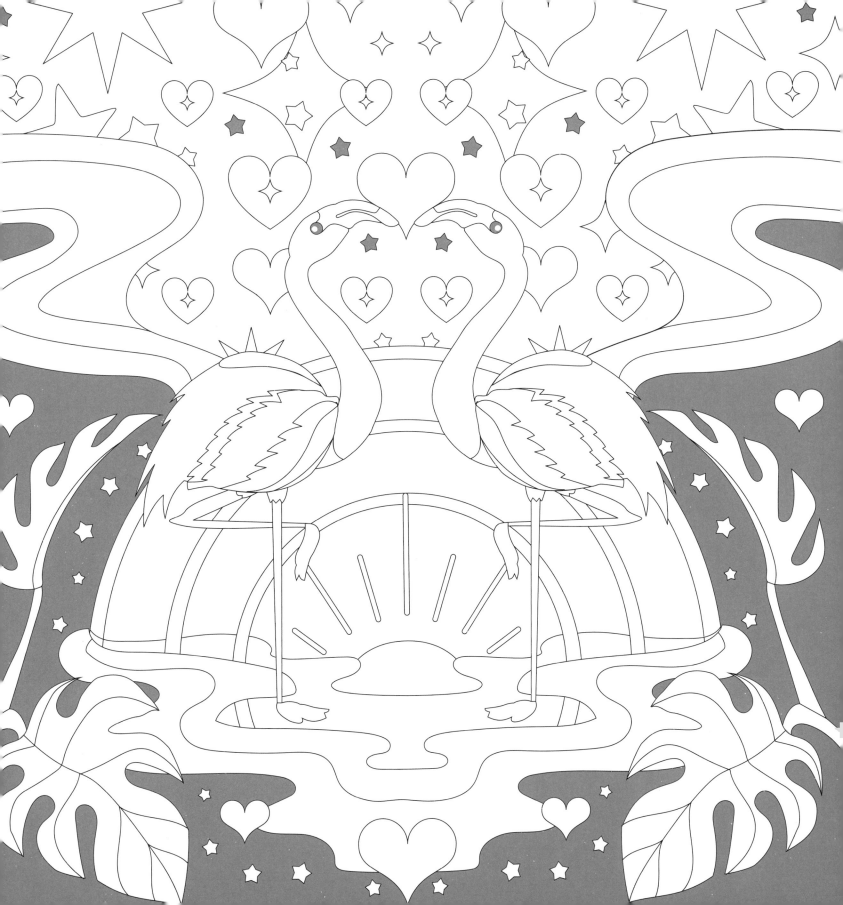

*Friendships are important to me.
I am creating a circle of positive,
uplifting friends who know and love
the real me. I let go of those who hold
me back or who no longer bring joy
into my life while acknowledging any
lessons I have learned from them.*

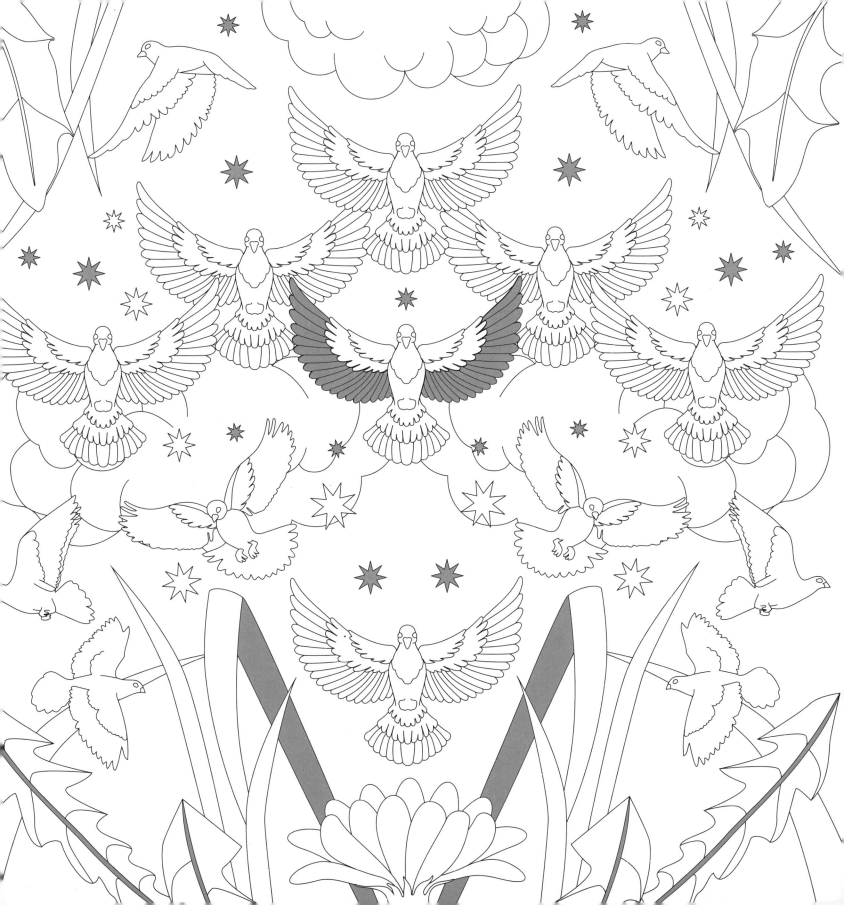

*I appreciate the deep roots of love already in my life from the people I choose to be connected to.
I am finding new ways to create intimacy and value in the relationships that are important to me as well as opening up to new connections.*

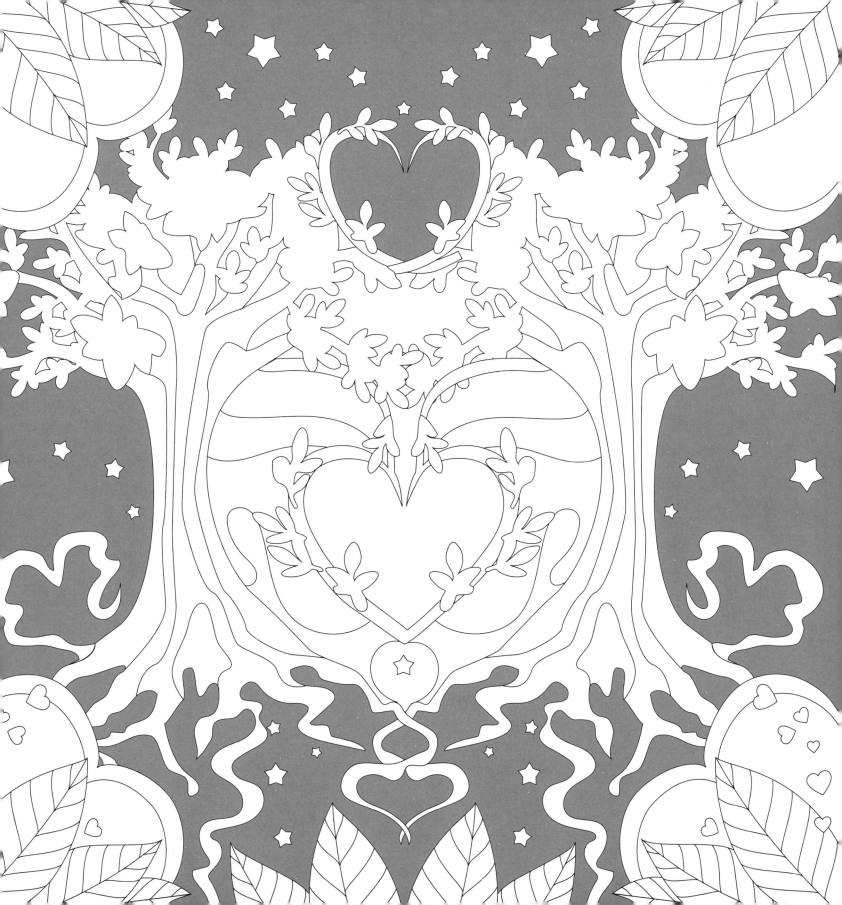

*I release past hurts and forgive those
who have hurt me as much as I am
able to. I forgive myself for harm
I have done to others and to myself.
I allow myself to move forward from
where I am now, knowing that
I am doing my best in all that I do.*

*There is nothing I need
to prove to others: I am strong
enough, loving enough,
and successful enough just
as I am. I am the best judge
of what is right for me.*

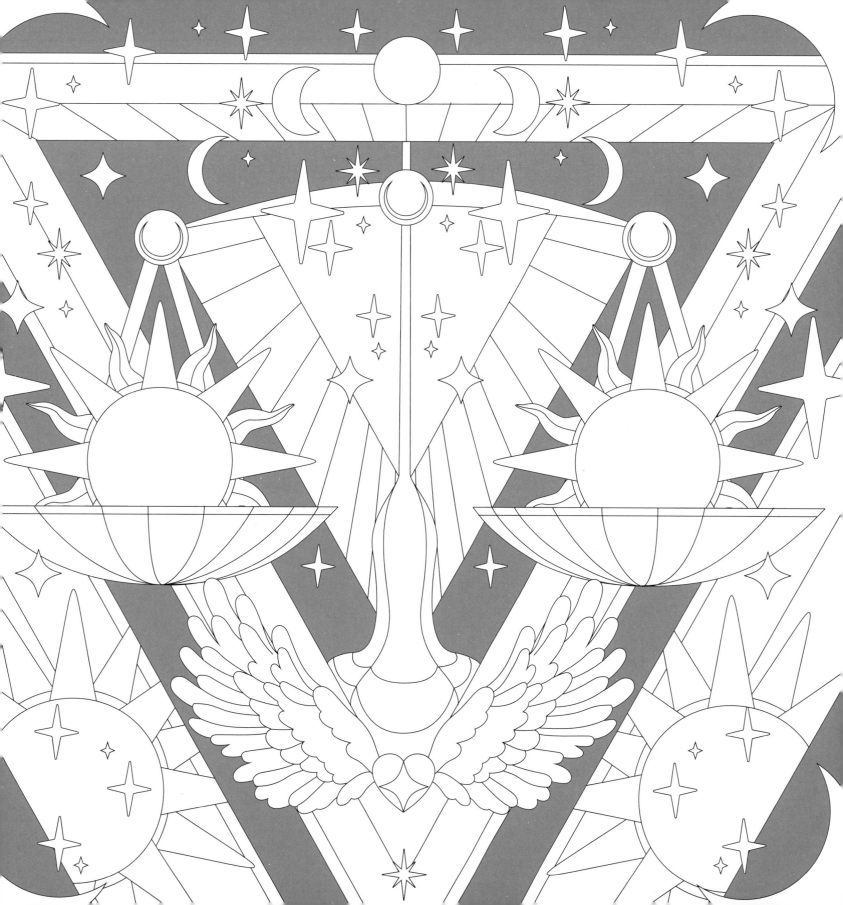

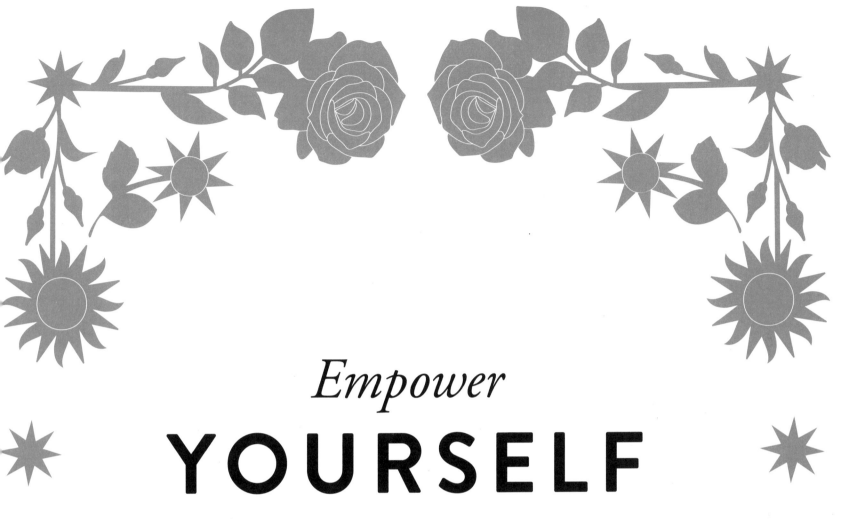

Empower

YOURSELF

Each morning I wake up
feeling happy and full
of energy for the day.

I love that I feel comfortable in my skin. It glows with health and has natural healing powers.

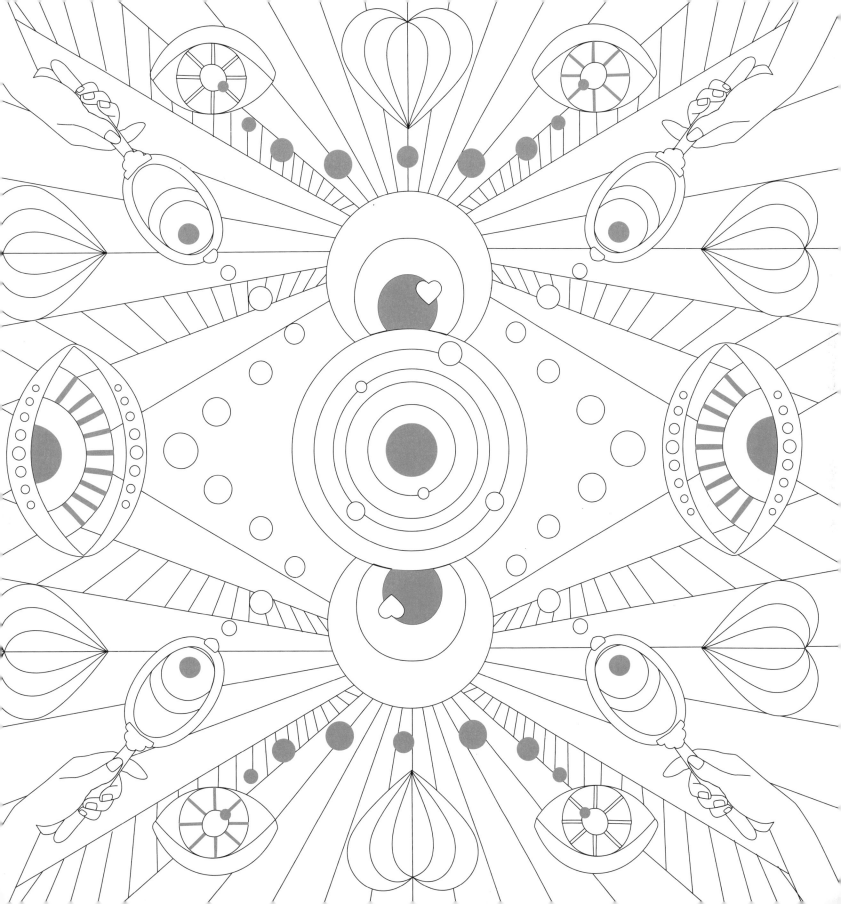

My body is beautiful just as it is. I am so grateful for all that it does for me and always treat it with kindness.

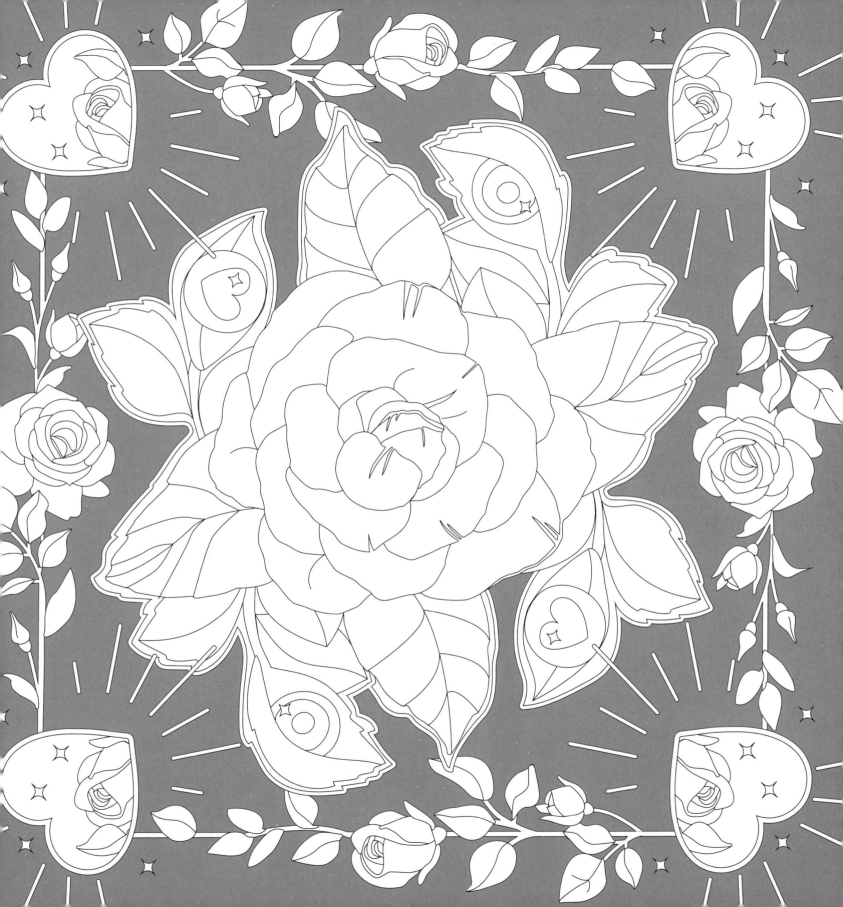

Exercise makes me feel happier, and I am getting fitter and stronger. I am in tune with my body's needs and allow myself rest days when I need them.

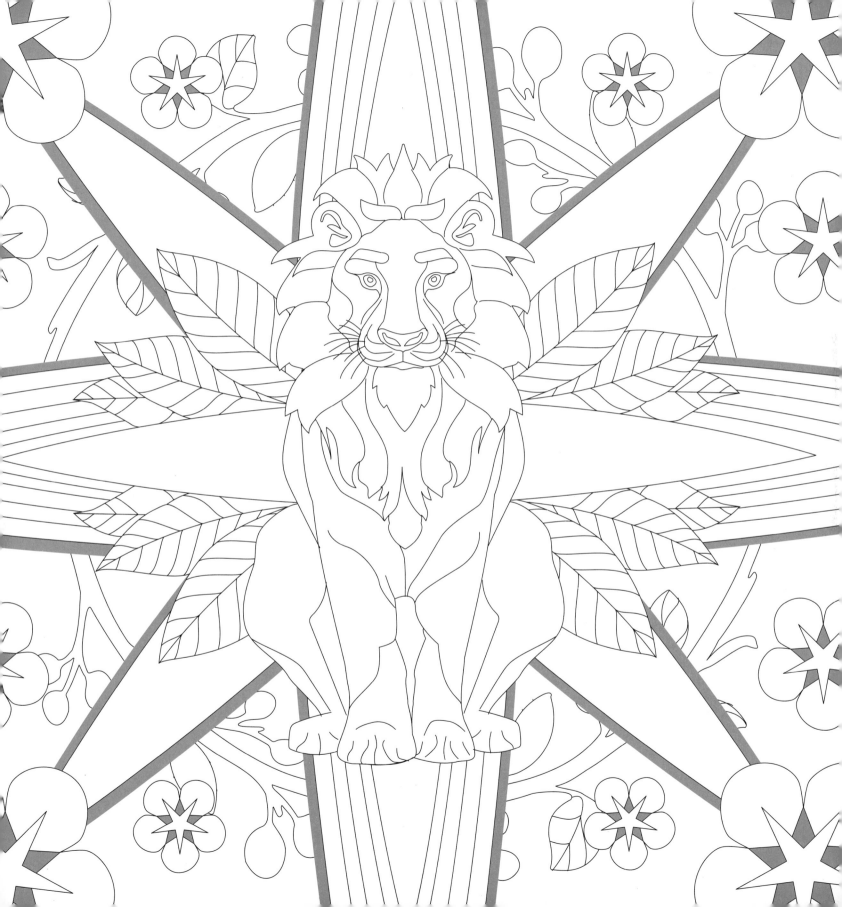

At night I access deep rest, knowing that the universe is aligning in my favor while I sleep.

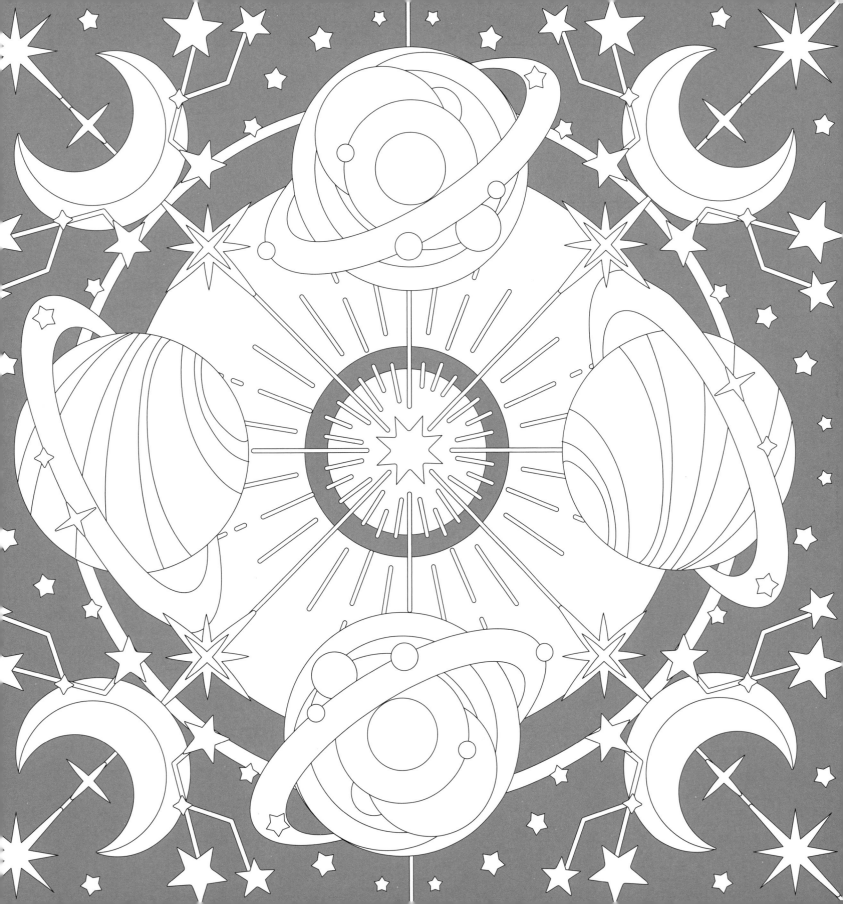

My home is becoming
a beautiful and calm space
to be in. It nurtures and supports me.
This is a place where I can relax and
recharge whenever I need to.

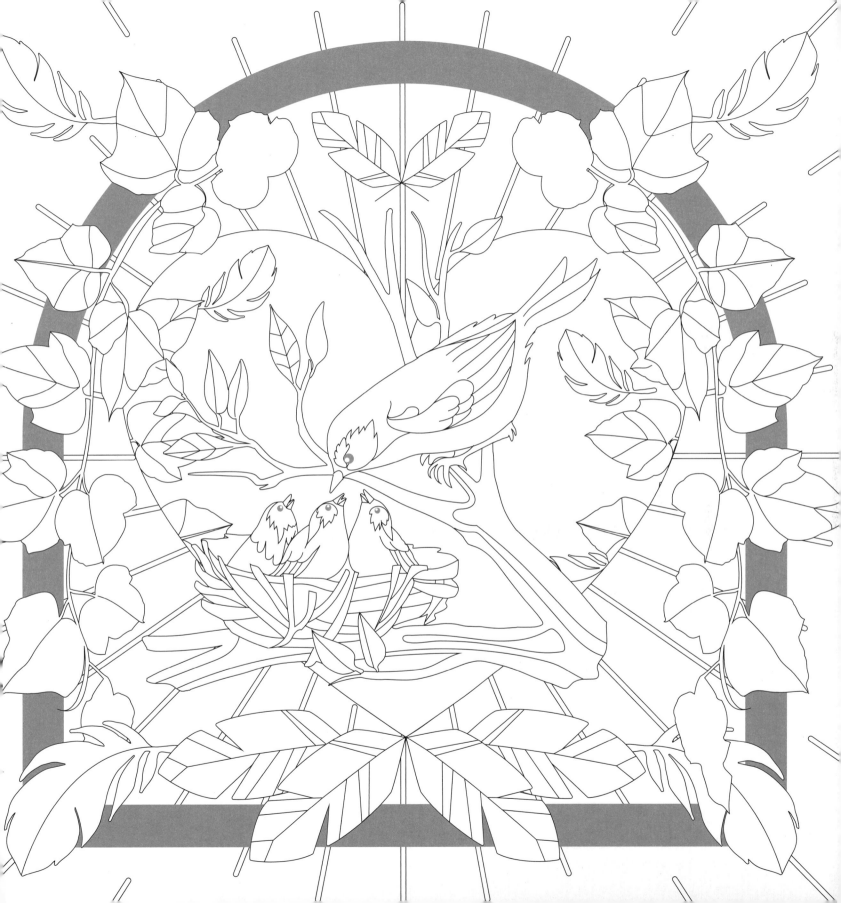

I am overflowing with joy and motivation today. I release habits that I want to change and take the steps to enable me to embrace a happier, healthier life.

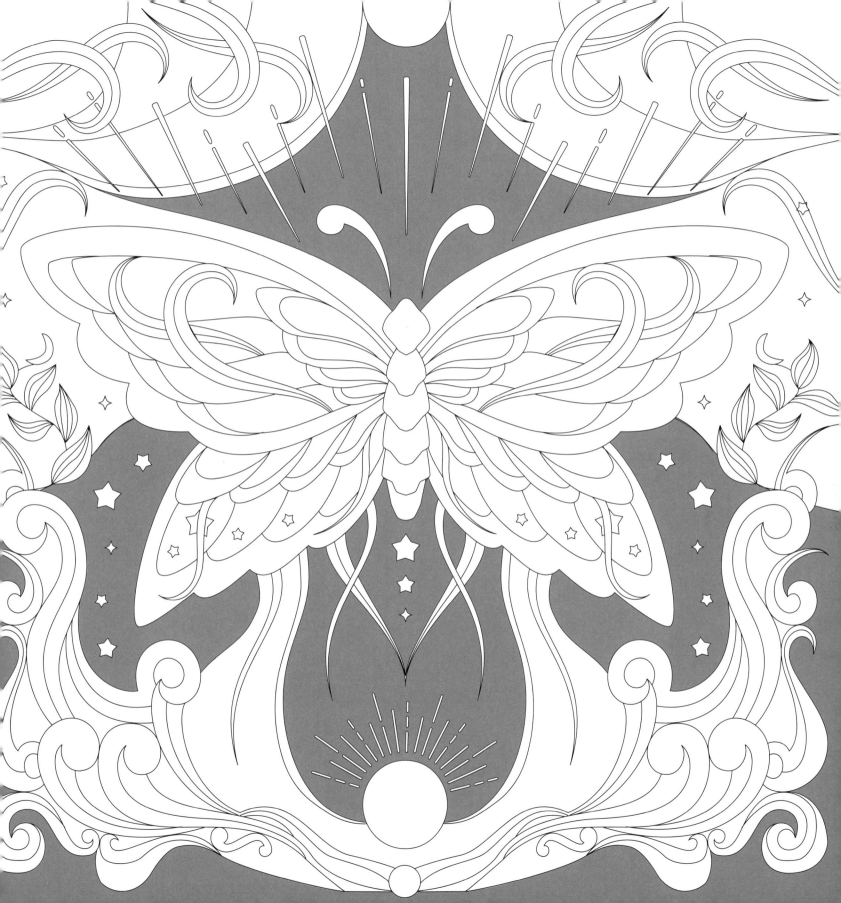

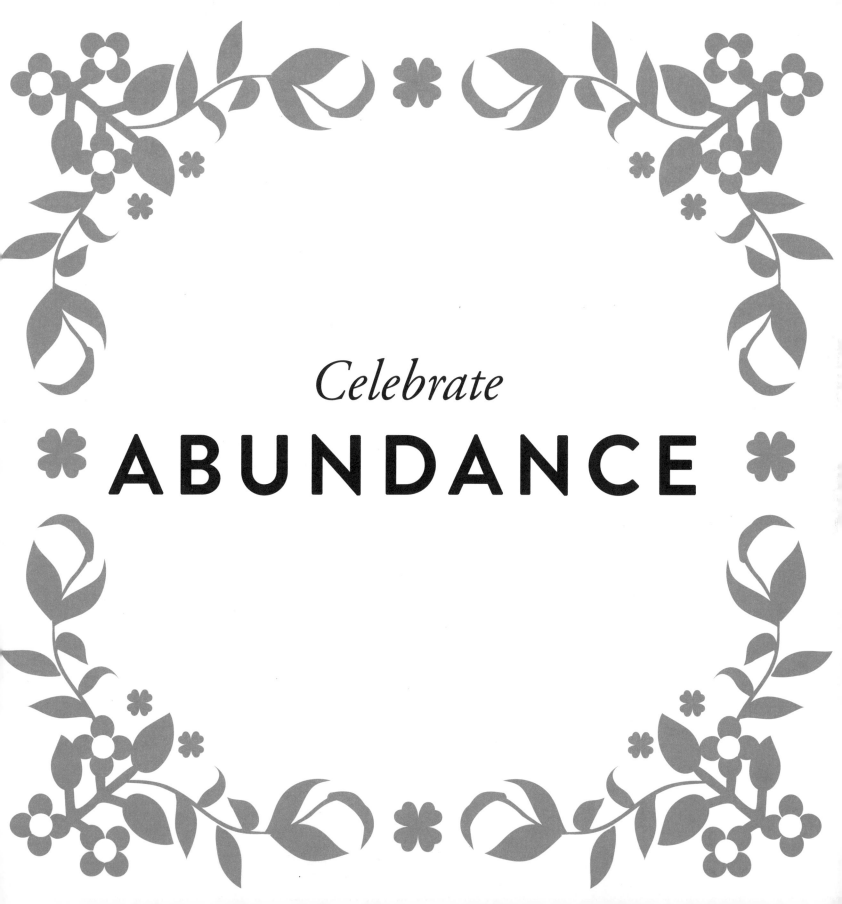

Celebrate

ABUNDANCE

I choose to be happy.
Everything I need is
already within my life
and I make the most
of all the opportunities
I am given.

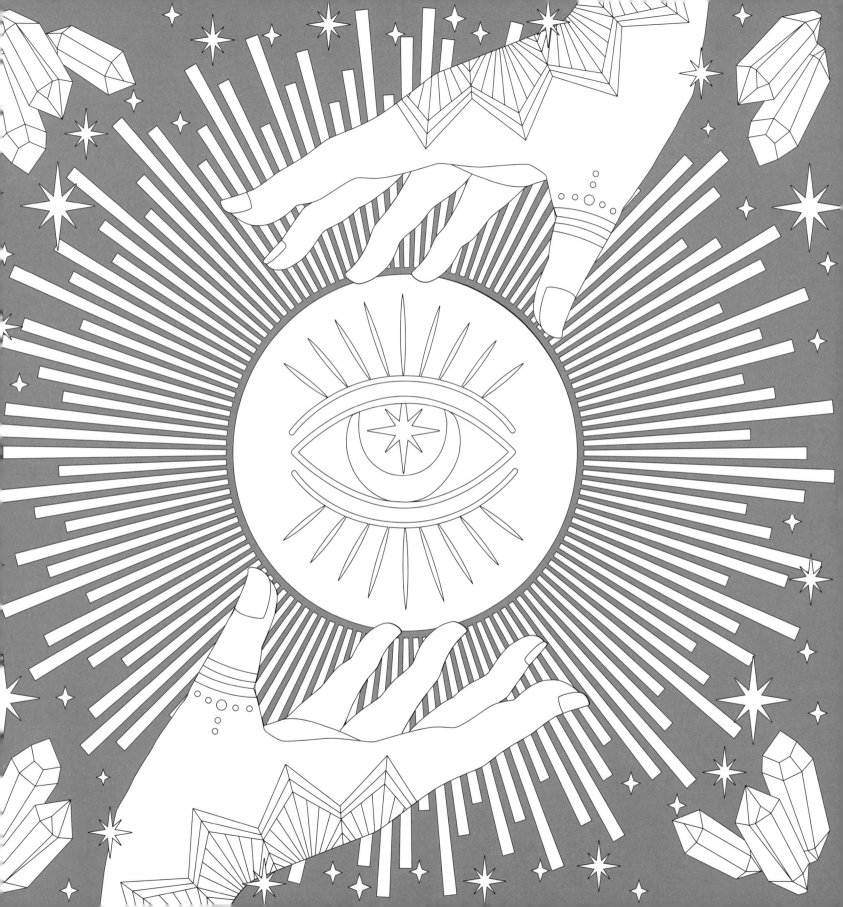

Everything I want is coming to fruition. I sow the seeds of my dream life every single day.

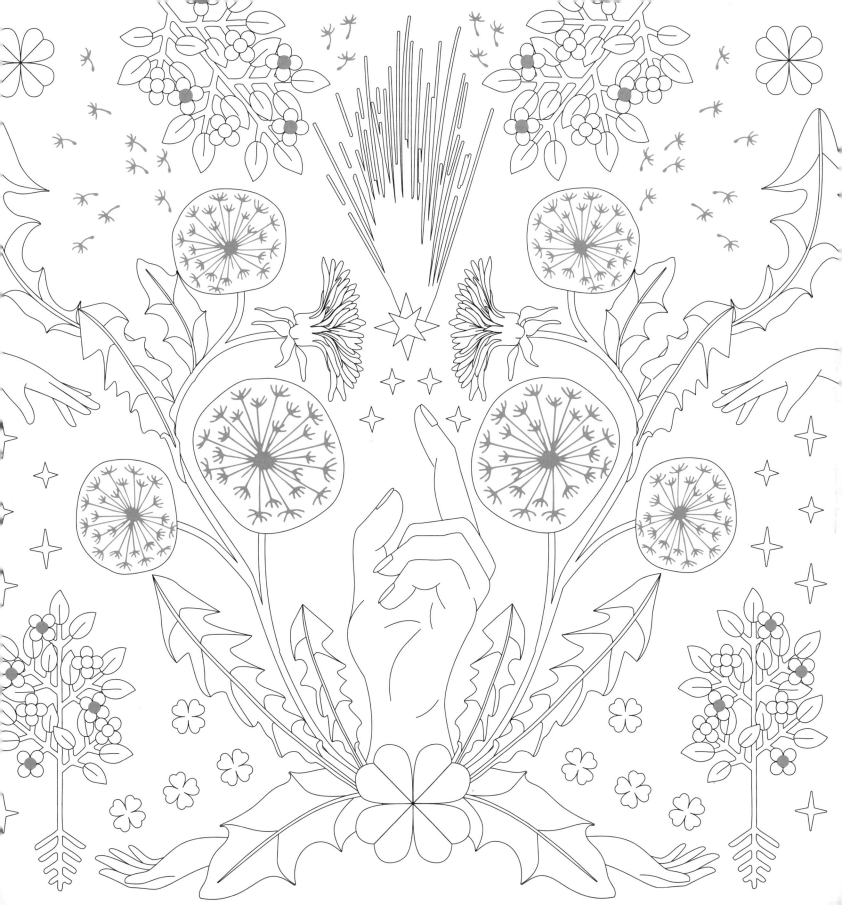

This world is a magical place. I draw inspiration from it and play my part in taking care of the beautiful planet we live in. I live in harmony with nature.

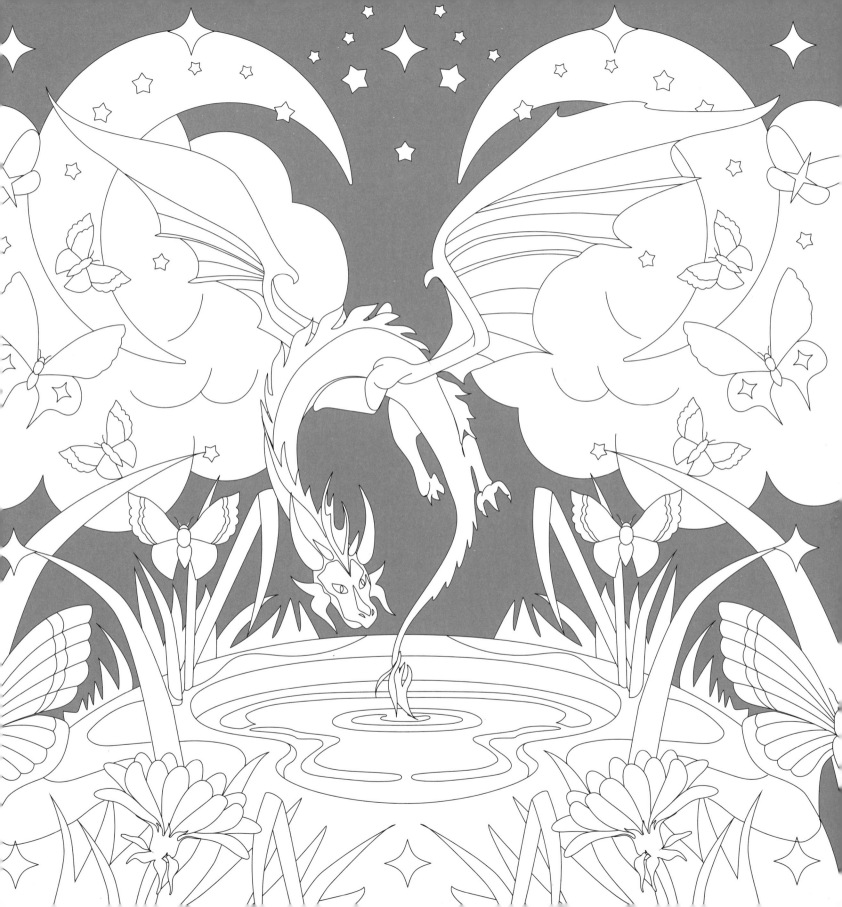

I let go of everything that limits me and I embrace the life I deserve.

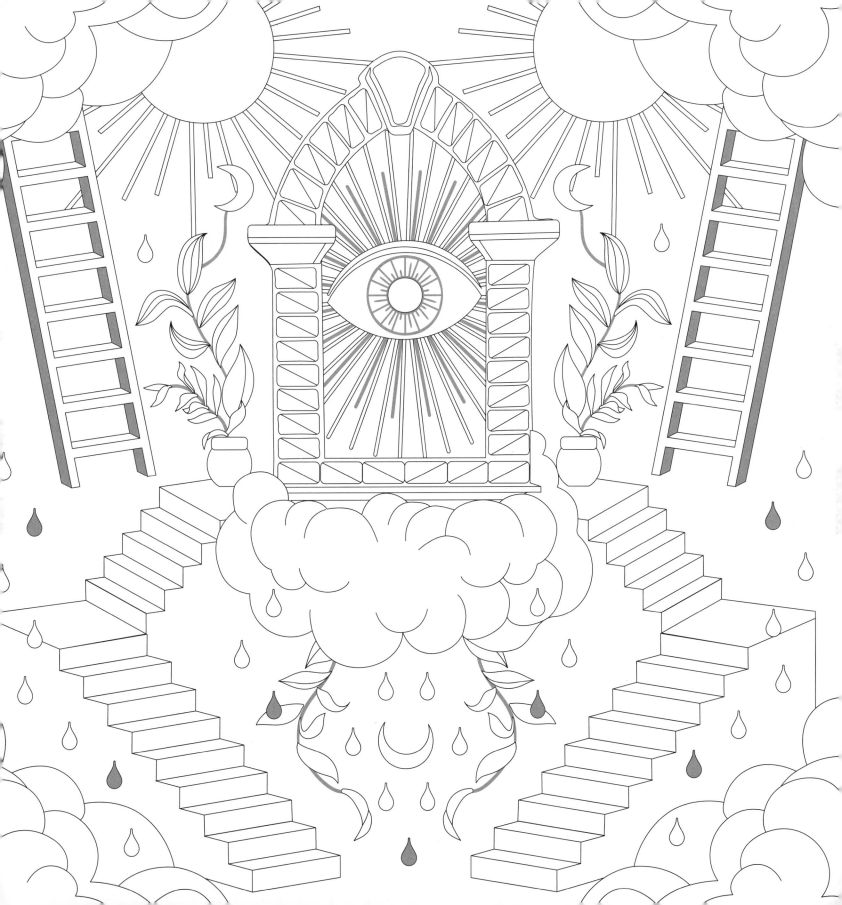

My capacity for love is limitless. I care for myself and those around me, and I also extend warm wishes outward to all beings.

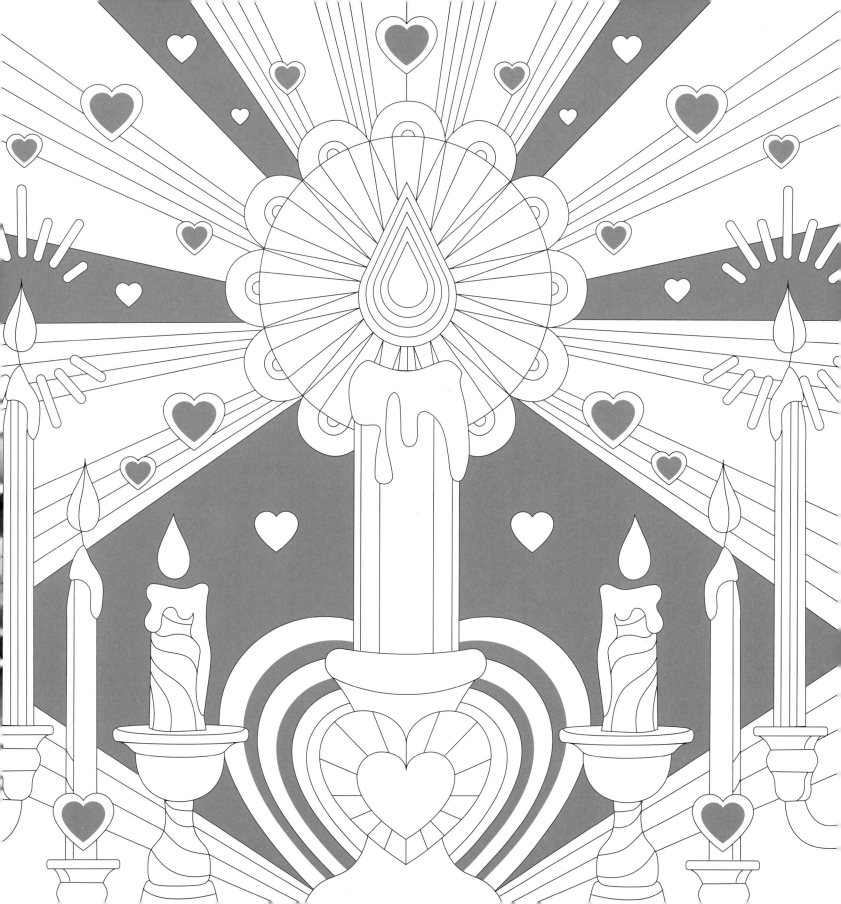